SALAD sync

SALA

SALAD SYNC IS A SALAD CHART WITH A

SALADS FILLED WITH AN ARRAY OF TEXTURE AND

USE THIS CHART TO BUILD NOURISHING

SALAD MADE EASY, FOLLOW THE CHART STEPS AND

sync©

SPRINKLE OF LOVE

WONDERFUL COLORS AND FRAGRANCES

YUMMY SALADS

VOILA ! YOUR SALAD IS READY !

ENJOY CREATING

FLAVORS THAT DANCE AROUND EACH OTHER

Celebrate the food and enjoy the flavor, taste, smell, look, texture, composition and design

The power of a salad can be a source of physical and mental wellness, positive energy and ongoing vitality

DELICIOUSNESS

SaladSync touches a little bit on the how, what, when and how we eat

SIMPLICITY & BALANCE

Building a Salad is easy.
Follow the Chart steps and
Voilà your salad is ready !

ENERGY

Enjoy a refreshing salad anytime

rapides à préparer

TABLEAU

Assembler votre salad.
Le choix est infini.

pour une salade

APPÉTISSANT

Salades des couleurs, textures et des saveurs

SALADSYNC ©

Collard & OR Chard	Squash	Tofu & OR Seitan	Corn & OR Pepper	Carrot & OR Onion	Sunflower seeds & OR Wallnuts	Tahini OR Asian dressing
Iceberg & OR Cabbage	Rice	Eggplant & OR Yam	Pea & OR Jicama	Avocado & OR Zucchini	Chestnuts OR Pecans	Thai Almond Butter OR Soy Sauce
Parsley	Couscous	Mushroom & OR Artichoke	Asparagus & OR Turnip	Tomato & OR Celery & OR Rutabaga	Sesame seeds & OR Brazil nuts	Pesto OR Mango Cilantro dressing
my favorite Lettuce	Pasta	Bean	Pomegranate & OR Parsnip	Cucumber & OR Radish & OR Daikon	Almonds & OR Edible flower	Chili Lime OR Soy Garlic dressing
Mixed Greens	Lentil	Jackfruit OR Tempeh	Okra & OR Brocoli	Papaya & OR Apple & OR Grapes	Pumpkin seeds & OR Crunchy Nutritional Yeast	Squeeze Lemon Salt, Pepper & Oil & OR My favorite Herb
Romaine Lettuce	Quinoa	Garbanzo Chickpea	String bean & OR Bok choy	Pear & OR Berries	unsweetened shredded Coconut & OR Pine seeds	Balsamic dressing OR Vegan Ranch OR Creamy Mustard
Kale	Grain	Potato & OR Cauliflower	Beet & OR Sprouts	my favorite Fruit	Chia seeds & OR my favorite Nuts	Cilantro Vinaigrette OR Garlic Ginger dressing

BUILDING MY SALAD RAINBOW ONE COLUMN AT A TIME

1st ingredient(s) from column 1
2nd ingredient(s) from column 2
3rd ingredient(s) from column 3
4th ingredient(s) from column 4
5th ingredient(s) from column 5
6th ingredient(s) from column 6
7th ingredient(s) from column 7

EACH COLUMN HAS
SEVEN SQUARES

SELECT ONE SQUARE
FROM EACH COLUMN

ONE page CHART CONTAINING AN

ABUNDANT

AMOUNT OF COMBINATIONS

Wow!

PRE PREPARE SOME OF THE INGREDIENTS IN YOUR FAVORITE STYLE

Some of the Chart ingredients are available in many types and many colors. Select any type and any color. Savor the different possibilities.

Ingredients in Perfect Harmony

tips

TO GET ALL THE BENEFITS A PLANT-BASED DIET OFFERS.

USE HEALTHY COOKING METHODS

Switch the item you picked to another if you have food restrictions or if it's not available at the market

- Dressing: Start with a small amount, increase for added flavor and preferred texture
- Wash your vegetables carefully
- Consider raw, sautéing, steaming, grilled, roast, boiling etc.
- Mince Dice Slice Shred etc..your Veggies & Fruits
- Oil: keep it low in saturated fats
- Dried Beans, Rice & Grains: Soak in water overnight
- Some Nuts should be soaked for 2 hours, & ideally overnight

PICK 100% WHOLE GRAINS

fun

Close your eyes & point to one square from each column.

No matter which square you pick from each column, the salad will turn out fantastic !

ideas

Copy Print the Chart on card-stock,

keep it with you while food shopping

Use the Chart as a placemat for your family and friends to create different combinations

BON
Appetit

SaladSync©

HOPES TO INSPIRE YOU TO CREATE YOUR OWN COMBINATIONS
WITH INGREDIENTS BEYOND THOSE ON THE CHART

SALAD

sync©

WITH A SPRINKLE OF

LOVE

SALAD SYNC IS DEDICATED TO
THE SENSES

some of these senses are

ELEMENTS

EARTH, FIRE, AIR, WATER & SPIRIT

EARTH FIRE WATER METAL & WOOD

FLAVORS

SWEET, SALTY, BITTER, SOUR, & UMAMI

TEXTURES

CRISP-JUICY, TOASTY-CRUNCHY & SOFT-CREAMY

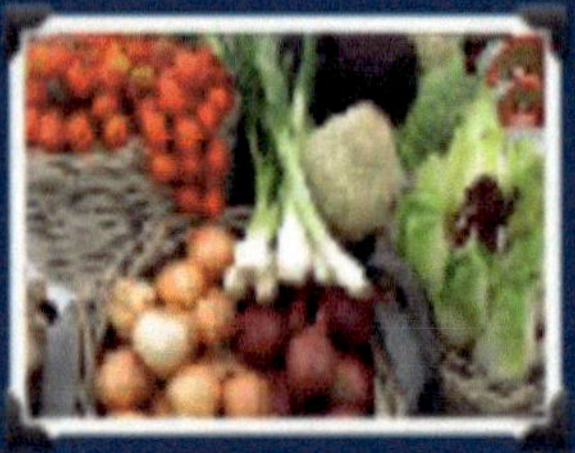

HAVE FUN USING THE SALAD SYNC CHART.

ENJOY A SALAD THAT IS EASY TO BUILD, AND DELICIOUS, NUTRITIOUS, LIGHT & CLEANSING, AND THAT OFFERS A SATISFYING JUXTAPOSITION OF TEXTURES.

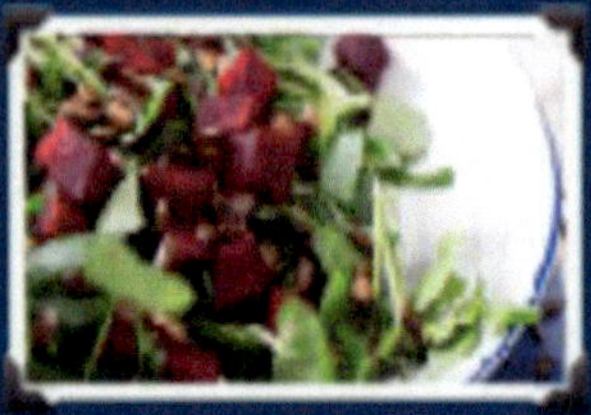

1st ingredient(s) from column 1
2nd ingredient(s) from column 2
3rd ingredient(s) from column 3
4th ingredient(s) from column 4
5th ingredient(s) from column 5
6th ingredient(s) from column 6
7th ingredient(s) from column 7

Refer to the CHART & the TIPS page.

Made in the USA
Monee, IL
05 November 2026

67386148R00017